The Complete Keto Diet Dishes Recipe Collection

Effortless Low Carb Recipes on a Budget To Lose Weight

Rebecca Marshall

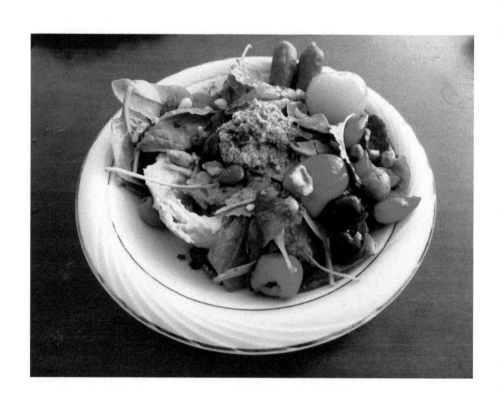

By reading this document, the reader agrees that under no circumstances is the author responsible for any losses, direct or indirect, which are incurred as a result of the use of information contained within this document, including, but not limited to, — errors, omissions, or inaccuracies.

Table of contents

Basic Keto Low Carb Chaffle Recipe

Preparation time: 10 minutes

Cooking Time: 8 Minutes

Servings: 2

Ingredients:

- 1 egg
- 1/2 cup cheddar cheese, shredded

Directions:

1. Turn Chaffle maker on or plug it in so that it heats and grease both sides.
2. In a small bowl, crack an egg, then add the 1/cup cheddar cheese and stir to combine.
3. Pour 1/2 of the batter in the Chaffle maker and close the top.
4. Cooking for 3-minutes or until it reaches desired doneness.
5. Carefully remove from Chaffle maker and set aside for 2-3 minutes to give it time to crisp.
6. Follow the Directions again to make the second chaffle.

Nutrition:

Calories: 58

Fat: 0.4g

Carbohydrates: 0g

Protein: 1.4g

Keto Avocado Chaffle Toast

Preparation time: 5 minutes

Cooking Time: 8 Minutes

Servings: 2

Ingredients:

Avocado Topping:

- 1 tbsp. butter
- 1 green bell pepper (finely chopped)
- 1/2 cup feta cheese
- 1/2 avocado
- 1 tsp. lemon juice
- 1/4 tsp. nutmeg
- 1/4 tsp. onion powder
- 1/2 tsp. ground black pepper or to taste

Chaffle:

- 1/2 mozzarella cheese
- 1 egg (beaten)
- 1 tbsp. Almond flour
- 1 tsp. cinnamon
- 1/2 tsp. baking soda

Directions:

1. Plug the Chaffle maker tom preheats it and spray it with a non-stick spray.

2. In a mixing bowl, combine the mozzarella, almond flour, baking soda and cinnamon. Add the egg and mix until the ingredients are well combined and you form a smooth batter.

3. Fill the Chaffle maker with appropriate amount of the batter and spread the batter to the edges of the Chaffle maker to cover all the holes on the Chaffle iron.

4. Close the lid of the Chaffle maker and Cooking for about 3 to minutes or according to Chaffle maker's settings.

5. Meanwhile, dice the avocado into a bowl and mash until smooth. Add the bell pepper, nutmeg, onion powder, ground pepper and lemon juice. Mix until well combined.

6. After the baking cycle, remove the chaffle the Chaffle maker with a silicone or plastic utensil.

7. Repeat step 3, 4 and 6 until you have cooked all the batter into chaffles.

8. Brush the butter over the chaffles. Spread the avocado mixture over the chaffles. Top with shredded feta cheese.

9. Serve and enjoy.

Nutrition:

Calories: 12

Fat: 10g

Carbohydrates: 5g

Protein: 1.2g

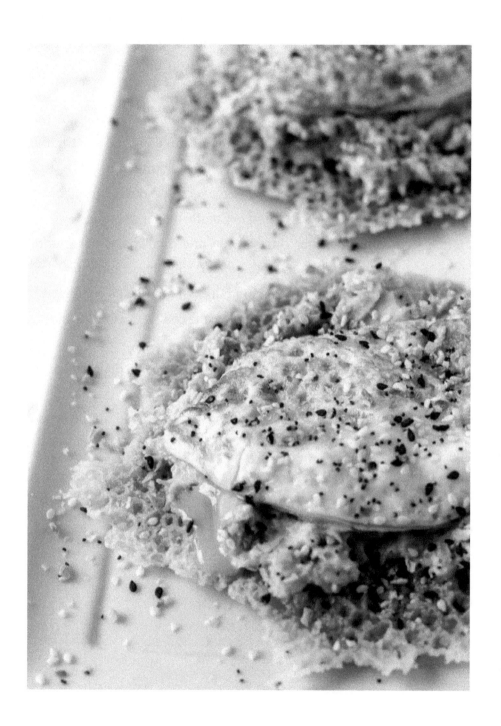

Okonomiyaki Style Chaffle

Preparation time: 5 minutes

Cooking Time: 8 Minutes

Servings: 2

Ingredients:

- 4 tbsp. finely shredded cabbage
- 2 eggs (beaten)
- 1/3 cup shredded mozzarella cheese
- 1 slice of bacon (finely chopped)
- A pinch of salt
- 1 tsp. tamari sauce
- 1 tbsp. chopped green onion
- 1/8 tsp. ground black pepper or to taste

Topping:

- 1 tbsp. kewpie mayonnaise or American mayonnaise
- 2 tbsp. bonito flakes
- 2 tsp. Worcestershire sauce

Directions:

1. Heat up a frying pan over medium to high heat and add the chopped bacon.
2. Sear until the bacon is brown and crispy. Use a slotted spoon to transfer the bacon to a paper towel lined plate to drain.
3. Plug the Chaffle maker to preheat it and spray it with a non-stick spray.

11

4. In a mixing bowl, combine the crispy bacon, cabbage, cheese, onion, pepper and salt. Add the egg and tamari. Mix until the ingredients are well combined.

5. Pour an appropriate amount of the batter into the Chaffle maker and spread out the batter to cover all the holes on the Chaffle maker.

6. Close the Chaffle maker and Cooking for about 4 minutes or according to your Chaffle maker's settings.

7. After the Cooking cycle, use a silicone or plastic utensil to remove the chaffle from the Chaffle maker.

8. Repeat step 5 to 7 until you have cooked all the batter into chaffles.

9. Top the chaffles with sauce, mayonnaise and bonito flakes.

10. Serve warm and enjoy.

Nutrition:

Calories: 167

Fat: 15g

Carbohydrates: 2.1g,

Protein: 5.2g

Zucchini Chaffles On Pan

Preparation time: 5 minutes

Cooking Time: 5 Minutes

Servings: 4

Ingredients:

- 1 cup zucchini, grated
- 1 egg
- 1 cup cheddar cheese
- pinch of salt
- 1 tbsp. avocado oil

Directions:

1. Heat your nonstick pan over medium heat.
2. Pour salt over grated zucchini and let it sit for 5 minutes Utes.
3. Remove water from zucchini
4. In a small bowl, mix zucchini, egg, and cheese together.
5. Grease pan with avocado oil.
6. Once the pan is hot, pour 2 tbsps. zucchini batter and Cooking for about 1-2 minutes Utes.
7. Flip and Cooking for another 1-2 minutes Utes.
8. Once the chaffle is brown, remove from pan.
9. Serve coconut cream on top and enjoy.

Nutrition:

Calories: 297

Fat: 14g

Carbohydrates: 15g

Protein: 15g

BLT Chaffle Sandwich

Preparation time: 5 minutes

Cooking Time: 10 Minutes

Servings: 2

Ingredients:

- Sandwich Filling:
- 2 strips of bacon
- A pinch of salt
- 2 slices tomato
- 1 tbsp. mayonnaise
- 3 pieces lettuce

Chaffle:

- 1 egg (beaten)
- 1/2 cup shredded mozzarella cheese
- 1/4 tsp. onion powder
- 1/4 tsp. garlic powder
- 1/2 tsp. curry powder

Directions:

1. Plug the Chaffle maker and preheat it. Spray it with a non-stick spray.
2. In a mixing bowl, combine the cheese, onion powder, garlic and curry powder. Add the egg and mix until the ingredients are well combined.

3. Fill the Chaffle maker with the batter and spread the batter to the edges of the Chaffle maker to cover all the holes on the Chaffle iron.

4. Close the lid of the Chaffle maker and Cooking for about minutes or according to Chaffle maker's settings.

5. After the Cooking cycle, remove the chaffle from the Chaffle maker using a silicone or plastic utensil.

6. Repeat step 3 to 5 until you have cooked all the batter into chaffles. Set the chaffles aside to cool.

7. Heat up a skillet over medium heat. Add the bacon strips and sear until all sides of the bacon is browned, turning and pressing the bacon while searing.

8. Use a slotted spoon to transfer the bacon to a paper towel lined plate to drain.

9. Place the chaffles on a flat surface and spread mayonnaise over the face of the chaffles.

10. Divide the lettuce into two and layer it on one portion on both chaffles.

11. Layer the tomatoes on one of the chaffles and sprinkle with salt. Layer the bacon over the tomatoes and place the other chaffle over the one containing the bacon.

12. Press and serve immediately. Enjoy!!!

Nutrition:

Calories: 130

Fat: 5g

Carbohydrates: 7g

Protein: 16g

Keto Chaffle Sandwich

Preparation time: 10 minutes

Cooking Time: 6 Minutes

Servings: 2

Ingredients:

- 1 egg
- 1/2 cup Monterey Jack Cheese
- 1 tablespoon almond flour
- 2 tablespoons butter

Directions:

1. In a small bowl, mix the egg, almond flour, and Monterey Jack Cheese.
2. Pour half of the batter into your mini Chaffle maker and Cooking for 3-4 minutes. Then Cooking the rest of the batter to make a second chaffle.
3. In a small pan, melt 2 tablespoons of butter. Add the chaffles and Cooking on each side for 2 minutes. Pressing down while they are Cooking lightly on the top of them, so they crisp up better.
4. Remove from the pan and let sit for 2 minutes.

Nutrition:

Calories: 152

Fat: 10g,

Carbohydrates: 4g

Protein: 4g

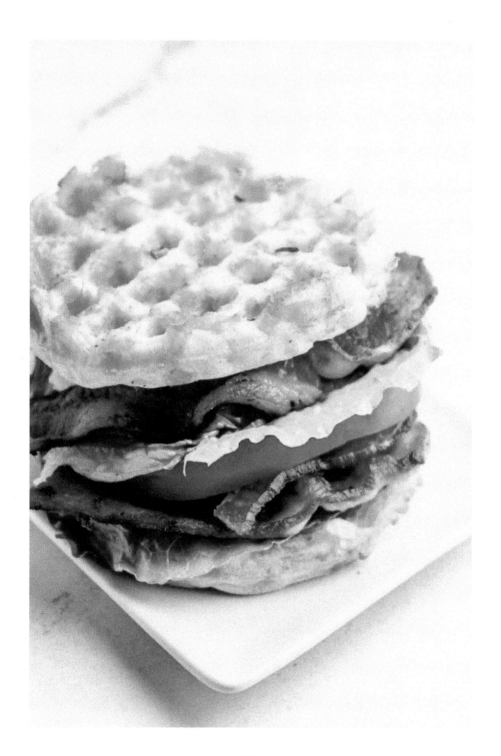

Cinnamon Rolls Chaffles

Preparation time: 10 minutes

Cooking Time: 10 Minutes

Servings: 2

Ingredients:

Cinnamon Roll Chaffle

- 1/2 cup mozzarella cheese
- 1 tablespoon almond flour
- 1/4 tsp. baking powder
- 1 egg
- 1 tsp. cinnamon
- 1 tsp. Granulated Swerve

Cinnamon roll swirl

- 1 tbsp. butter
- 1 tsp. cinnamon
- 2 tsp. confectioner's swerve

Keto Cinnamon Roll Glaze

- 1 tablespoon butter
- 1 tablespoon cream cheese
- 1/4 tsp. vanilla extract
- 2 tsp. swerve confectioners

Directions:

1. Plug in your Mini Dash Chaffle maker and let it heat up.

2. In a small bowl mix the mozzarella cheese, almond flour, baking powder, egg, 1 teaspoon cinnamon, and 1 teaspoon swerve granulated and set aside.

3. In another small bowl, add a tablespoon of butter, 1 teaspoon cinnamon, and 2 teaspoons of swerve confectioners' sweetener.

4. Microwave for 15 seconds and mix well.

5. Spray the Chaffle maker with nonstick spray and add 1/3 of the batter to your Chaffle maker. Swirl in 1/3 of the cinnamon, swerve, and butter mixture onto the top of it. Close the Chaffle maker and let Cooking for 3-4 minutes.

6. When the first cinnamon rolls chaffle is done, make the second and then make the third.

7. While the third chaffle is Cooking place 1 tablespoon butter and 1 tablespoon of cream cheese in a small bowl. Heat in the microwave for 10-15 seconds. Start at 10, and if the cream cheese is not soft enough to mix with the butter heat for an additional 5 seconds.

8. Add the vanilla extract and the swerve confectioner's sweetener to the butter and cream cheese and mix well using a whisk.

9. Drizzle keto cream cheese glaze on top of chaffle.

Nutrition:

Calories: 302

Fat: 28g

Carbohydrates: 4g

Protein: 9g

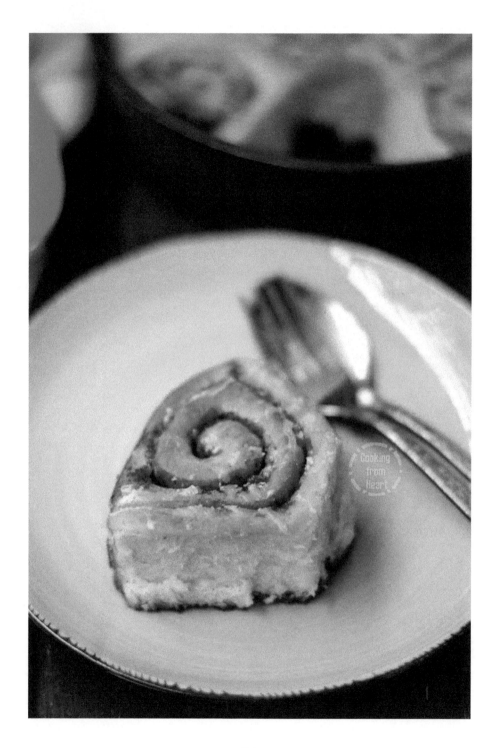

Chocolate Chip Chaffle Keto

Preparation time: 10 minutes

Cooking Time: 8 Minutes

Servings: 2

Ingredients:

- 1 egg
- 1 tbsp. heavy whipping cream
- 1/2 tsp. coconut flour
- 1 3/4 tsp. Lakanto monk fruit golden can use more or less to adjust sweetness
- 1/4 tsp. baking powder
- pinch of salt
- 1 tbsp. Lily's Chocolate Chips

Directions:

1. Turn on the Chaffle maker device.
2. In a small bowl, merge all ingredients except the chocolate chips and stir well until combined.
3. Grease Chaffle maker, and then pour half of the batter onto the bottom plate of the Chaffle maker. Sprinkle a few chocolate chips on top and then close.
4. Cook for 3-minutes or until the chocolate chip chaffle dessert is golden brown, then detach from Chaffle maker with a fork, being careful not to burn your fingers.
5. Repeat with the rest of the batter.

6. Let chaffle sit for a few minutes so that it begins to crisp.

Nutrition:

Calories: 205

Fat: 19g,

Carbohydrates: g

Protein: 2.8g

Cheesy Garlic Chaffle Bread

Preparation time: 10 minutes

Cooking Time: 14 Minutes

Servings: 2

Ingredients:

- 1 egg
- 1/2 cup mozzarella cheese, shredded
- 1 tbsp. parmesan cheese
- 3/4 tsp. coconut flour
- 1/4 tsp. baking powder
- 1/8 tsp. Italian Seasoning
- Pinch of salt
- 1 tbsp. butter, melted
- 1/4 tsp. garlic powder
- 1/2 cup mozzarella cheese, shredded
- 1/4 tsp. basil seasoning

Directions:

1. Preheat oven to 400 degrees. Plug the Dash Mini Chaffle Maker in the wall and allow it to get hot. Lightly grease Chaffle maker.
2. Combine the first 7 ingredients in a small bowl and stir well to combine.
3. Spoon half of the batter on the Chaffle maker and close — Cooking for 4 minutes or until golden brown.

4. Remove the chaffle bread carefully from the Dash Mini Chaffle Maker, then repeat for the rest of the batter.
5. In a small bowl, melt the butter and add garlic powder.
6. Cut each chaffle in half (or thirds), and place on a baking sheet, then brush the tops with the garlic butter mixture.
7. Top with mozzarella cheese and pop in the oven for 4 -5 minutes.
8. Turn oven to broil and move the baking pan to the top shelf for 1-2 minutes so that the cheese begins to bubble and turn golden brown. Watch very carefully, as it can burn quickly on broil. (check every 30 seconds)
9. Remove from oven and sprinkle basil seasoning on top. Enjoy!

Nutrition:

Calories: 85

Fat: 4g

Carbohydrates: 2g

Protein: 3g

Easy Keto Chaffle Sausage Gravy

Preparation time: 10 minutes

Cooking Time: 10 Minutes

Servings: 2

Ingredients:

For the Chaffle:

- 1 egg
- 1/2 cup mozzarella cheese, grated
- 1 tsp. coconut flour
- 1 tsp. water
- 1/4 tsp. baking powder
- Pinch of salt

For the Keto Sausage Gravy:

- 1/4 cup breakfast sausage, browned
- 3 tbsp. chicken broth
- 2 tbsp. heavy whipping cream
- 2 tsp. cream cheese, softened
- Dash garlic powder
- Pepper to taste
- Dash of onion powder (optional)

Directions:

1. Plug Dash Mini Chaffle Maker into the wall and allow it to heat up. Grease lightly or use Cooking spray.

2. Combine all the ingredients for the chaffle into a small bowl and stir to combine well.
3. Pour half of the chaffle batter onto the Chaffle maker, and then shut the lid and Cooking for approximately 4 minutes.
4. Remove chaffle from Chaffle maker and repeat the same process to make the second chaffle. Set aside to crisp.
5. Cooking one pound of breakfast sausage and drain. Reserve 1/4 cup for this recipe.

Nutrition:

Calories: 277

Fat: 21g

Carbohydrates: 7g

Protein: 10g

Keto Cheesy Garlic Bread Chaffle Recipe

Preparation time: 25 minutes

Cooking Time: 15 minutes

Serving: 2

Ingredients:

- Mozzarella cheese, one cup
- Eggs, two for adding into the chaffles
- Chopped fresh cilantro, 20 grams
- Butter, 34 grams
- Chopped garlic, 17 grams
- Salt to taste
- Italian seasoning, 17 grams
- Parmesan cheese, half cup

Directions:

1. Heat your Chaffle maker.
2. Always remember you heat your Chaffle maker till the point that it starts producing steam.
3. Remove the egg whites in a bowl and beat them to the point that they become fluffy.
4. Beat the egg yolks in a separate bowl.
5. Add in the egg yolks in the egg whites and delicately mix them with a spatula.
6. Combine the eggs and the rest of the ingredients except the chopped garlic, Italian seasoning, parmesan cheese, and the butter.

7. Add in the shredded chicken once the rest of the ingredients are well mixed.

8. When your Chaffle maker is heated adequately, pour in the mixture.

9. Close your Chaffle maker.

10. Let your chaffle Cooking for five to six minutes approximately.

11. When your chaffles are done, dish them out.

12. Mix the butter, chopped garlic and the Italian seasoning in a bowl.

13. Spread the butter mixture on the chaffles with the help of a brush.

14. Add the shredded parmesan cheese on top.

15. Your dish is ready to be served.

Nutrition:

Calories: 95

Fat: 5.8g

Carbohydrates: 2.2g

Sugar: 0.3g

Protein: 8g

Keto Jalapeno Popper Chaffle Recipe

Preparation time: 15 minutes

Cooking Time: 10 minutes

Serving: 2

Ingredients:

- Mozzarella cheese, one cup
- Eggs, two for adding into the chaffles
- Chopped fresh cilantro, 20 grams
- Cream cheese, 34 grams
- Salt to taste
- Italian seasoning, 17 grams
- Jalapeno poppers, half cup

Directions:

1. Heat your Chaffle maker.
2. Always remember you heat your Chaffle maker till the point that it starts producing steam.
3. Remove the egg whites in a bowl and beat them to the point that they become fluffy.
4. Beat the egg yolks in a separate bowl.
5. Add in the egg yolks in the egg whites and delicately mix them with a spatula.
6. Combine the eggs and the rest of the ingredients except the cream cheese and cilantro.
7. Add in the shredded chicken once the rest of the ingredients are well mixed.

8. When your Chaffle maker is heated adequately, pour in the mixture.
9. Close your Chaffle maker.
10. Let your chaffle Cooking for five to six minutes approximately.
11. When your chaffles are done, dish them out.
12. Add the cream cheese and cilantro on top.
13. Your dish is ready to be served.

Nutrition:

Calories: 99

Fat: 4.2g

Carbohydrates: 0.4g

Sugar: 0.2g

Protein: 5.7g

Keto Pumpkin Chaffle Recipe

Preparation time: 15 minutes

Cooking Time: 10 minutes

Serving: 2

Ingredients:

- Mozzarella cheese, one cup
- Eggs, two for adding into the chaffles
- Pumpkin spice, 17 grams
- Vanilla essence, 34 grams
- Baking powder, 17 grams
- Coconut flour, 34 grams
- Pumpkin puree, half cup
- Sugar free syrup, as required

Directions:

1. Heat your Chaffle maker.
2. Always remember you heat your Chaffle maker till the point that it starts producing steam.
3. Remove the egg whites in a bowl and beat them to the point that they become fluffy.
4. Beat the egg yolks in a separate bowl.
5. Add in the egg yolks in the egg whites and delicately mix them with a spatula.
6. Combine the eggs, cheese, spices, puree, coconut flour, vanilla essence, baking powder and coconut flour.

7. When your Chaffle maker is heated adequately, pour in the mixture.
8. Close your Chaffle maker.
9. Let your chaffle Cooking for five to six minutes approximately.
10. When your chaffles are done, dish them out.
11. Add sugar free syrup on top of the chaffles.
12. Your dish is ready to be served.

Nutrition:

Protein: 45

Fat: 47

Carbohydrates: 8

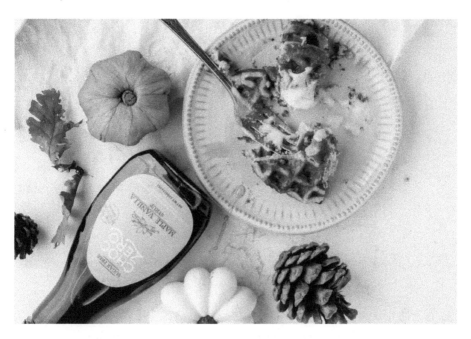

Keto Butter Chicken Chaffle with Tzatziki Sauce Recipe

Preparation time: 15 minutes

Cooking Time: 10 minutes

Serving: 2

Ingredients:

- Mozzarella cheese, one cup
- Eggs, two for adding into the chaffles
- Cheddar cheese, one cup
- Salt to taste
- Black pepper to taste
- Almond flour, 17 grams
- Shredded butter chicken, one cup
- Butter chicken sauce, half cup
- Tzatziki sauce, a quarter cup
- Chopped cilantro, 17 grams

Directions:

1. Heat your Chaffle maker.
2. Always remember you heat your Chaffle maker till the point that it starts producing steam.
3. Remove the egg whites in a bowl and beat them to the point that they become fluffy.
4. Beat the egg yolks in a separate bowl.
5. Add in the egg yolks in the egg whites and delicately mix them with a spatula.

6. Combine the eggs and the rest of the ingredients except the chicken, cilantro and tzatziki sauce.

7. Add in the shredded chicken once the rest of the ingredients are well mixed.

8. When your Chaffle maker is heated adequately, pour in the mixture.

9. Close your Chaffle maker.

10. Let your chaffle Cooking for five to six minutes approximately.

11. When your chaffles are done, dish them out.

12. Add the chopped cilantro on top of the chaffles.

13. You can also serve tzatziki sauce alongside your chaffles.

14. Your dish is ready to be served.

Nutrition:

Protein: 31

Fat: 66

Carbohydrates: 2

Keto Parmesan Garlic Chaffle Recipe

Preparation time: 15 minutes

Cooking Time: 10 minutes

Serving: 2

Ingredients:

- Mozzarella cheese, one cup
- Eggs, two for adding into the chaffles
- Chopped fresh cilantro, 20 grams
- Garlic powder, 17 grams
- Salt to taste
- Italian seasoning, 17 grams
- Parmesan cheese, half cup

Directions:

1. Heat your Chaffle maker.
2. Always remember you heat your Chaffle maker till the point that it starts producing steam.
3. Remove the egg whites in a bowl and beat them to the point that they become fluffy.
4. Beat the egg yolks in a separate bowl.
5. Add in the egg yolks in the egg whites and delicately mix them with a spatula.
6. Combine the eggs, cheese, garlic powder and salt.
7. Add in the shredded chicken once the rest of the ingredients are well mixed.

8. When your Chaffle maker is heated adequately, pour in the mixture.
9. Close your Chaffle maker.
10. Let your chaffle Cooking for five to six minutes approximately.
11. When your chaffles are done, dish them out.
12. Garnish it with a little parmesan and cilantro on top.
13. Your dish is ready to be served.

Nutrition:

Calories: 141

Fat: 8.9g

Carbohydrates: 1.1g

Sugar: 0.2g

Protein: 13.5g

Keto Roasted Beef Chaffle Sandwich Recipe

Preparation time: 20 minutes

Cooking Time: 15 minutes

Serving: 2

Ingredients:

- Mozzarella cheese, one cup
- Eggs, two for adding into the chaffles
- Mayonnaise, 34 grams
- Dijon mustard, 17 grams
- Salt to taste
- Black pepper to taste
- Beef, 50 grams
- Olive oil, 17 grams

Directions:

1. Heat your Chaffle maker.
2. Always remember you heat your Chaffle maker till the point that it starts producing steam.
3. Remove the egg whites in a bowl and beat them to the point that they become fluffy.
4. Beat the egg yolks in a separate bowl.
5. Add in the egg yolks in the egg whites and delicately mix them with a spatula.
6. Combine the eggs and the cheese as one.

7. When your Chaffle maker is heated adequately, pour in the mixture.
8. Close your Chaffle maker.
9. Let your chaffle Cooking for five to six minutes approximately.
10. In the meanwhile, Cooking your roast beef in a pan with olive oil.
11. Add in the salt and pepper on top of the eggs.
12. When done, dish them out on a plate.
13. Cut thin slices of roasted beef on top of your chaffle.
14. When your chaffles are done, dish them out.
15. Add on top of the chaffles a little mayonnaise, the Dijon mustard sauce and the roasted beef slice.
16. Make it a sandwich by placing another chaffle piece.
17. Your dish is ready to be served.

Nutrition:

Carbs: 3 g

Fat: 42 g

Protein: 34 g

Calories: 545

Keto Reuben Chaffle Sandwich Recipe

Preparation time: 15 minutes

Cooking Time: 10 minutes

Serving: 2

Ingredients:

- Mozzarella cheese, one cup
- Eggs, two for adding into the chaffles
- Swiss cheese, two slices
- Salt to taste
- Black pepper to taste
- Corned beef, 50 grams
- Sauerkraut, 50 grams
- Butter, 17 grams

Directions:

1. Heat your Chaffle maker.
2. Always remember you heat your Chaffle maker till the point that it starts producing steam.
3. Remove the egg whites in a bowl and beat them to the point that they become fluffy.
4. Beat the egg yolks in a separate bowl.
5. Add in the egg yolks in the egg whites and delicately mix them with a spatula.
6. Combine the eggs and the rest of the ingredients except the cheese slices, sauerkraut, and corned beef slices.

7. When your Chaffle maker is heated adequately, pour in the mixture.

8. Close your Chaffle maker.

9. Let your chaffle Cooking for five to six minutes approximately.

10. When your chaffles are done, dish them out.

11. Add a little butter in a pan and then add a piece of chaffle on top of the butter.

12. Lay a slice of corned beef, Swiss cheese and sauerkraut and place another chaffle piece on top.

13. Cooking your sandwich until the cheese melts by flipping it on both sides.

14. Your dish is ready to be served.

Nutrition:

Calories: 509

Carbohydrates: 5g

Fat: 45g

Protein: 23g

Keto Teri Avocado Chaffle Sandwich Recipe

Preparation time: 25 minutes

Cooking Time: 20 minutes

Serving: 2

Ingredients:

- Mozzarella cheese, one cup
- Eggs, two for adding into the chaffles
- For patties:
- Chopped fresh cilantro, 20 grams
- Egg, one
- Salt to taste
- Black pepper to taste
- Ground beef, half pound
- Pork rinds, 17 grams
- For garnish:
- Avocado slices, half cup
- Lettuce leaf, two
- For Teriyaki sauce:
- Soy sauce, 17 grams
- Japanese sake, 34 grams
- Swerve, 17 grams
- Xanthan gum, 5 grams

Directions:

1. Heat your Chaffle maker.
2. Always remember you heat your Chaffle maker till the point that it starts producing steam.
3. Remove the egg whites in a bowl and beat them to the point that they become fluffy.
4. Beat the egg yolks in a separate bowl.
5. Add in the egg yolks in the egg whites and delicately mix them with a spatula.
6. Combine the eggs and cheese for the chaffle.
7. When your Chaffle maker is heated adequately, pour in the mixture.
8. Close your Chaffle maker.
9. Let your chaffle Cooking for five to six minutes approximately.
10. When your chaffles are done, dish them out.
11. In the meanwhile, mix all the ingredients for the Teriyaki sauce in a bowl.
12. Mix the ingredients for the patties.
13. Make small two patties and fry them in olive oil until they are done.
14. Lay a lettuce leaf on the chaffle, add the patty and place the avocado slices on top.
15. Pour the teriyaki sauce on top and close your sandwich.
16. Your dish is ready to be served.

Nutrition:

Cal: 165

Total Fat 14 g

Saturated Fat 7 g

Cholesterol 632 mg

Sodium 497 mg

Keto Western Bacon Cheeseburger Chaffle Recipe

Preparation time: 25 minutes

Cooking Time: 20 minutes

Serving: 2

Ingredients:

- Mozzarella cheese, one cup
- Eggs, two for adding into the chaffles
- Chopped fresh cilantro, 20 grams
- Egg, one
- Salt to taste
- Black pepper to taste
- Ground beef burger patty, two
- Pork strips, four
- For garnish:
- Onion rings, four
- Cheddar cheese slices, two
- Sugar free barbeque sauce, 34 grams
- Olive oil, 17 grams

Directions:

1. Heat your Chaffle maker.
2. Always remember you heat your Chaffle maker till the point that it starts producing steam.

3. Remove the egg whites in a bowl and beat them to the point that they become fluffy.
4. Beat the egg yolks in a separate bowl.
5. Add in the egg yolks in the egg whites and delicately mix them with a spatula.
6. Combine the eggs and the rest of the ingredients for the chaffle.
7. When your Chaffle maker is heated adequately, pour in the mixture.
8. Close your Chaffle maker.
9. Let your chaffle Cooking for five to six minutes approximately.
10. When your chaffles are done, dish them out.
11. Fry the burger patty in olive oil until they are done.
12. Lay the burger patty on the chaffle.
13. Pour the sugar free barbeque sauce, and place the onion rings on top.
14. Close your sandwich.
15. Your dish is ready to be served.

Nutrition:

Calories 292

Fat 26g

Protein 14g

Carbs: 2.8

Keto Chaffle Crab Roll Recipe

Preparation time: 25 minutes

Cooking Time: 15 minutes

Serving: 2

Ingredients:

- Mozzarella cheese, one cup
- Eggs, two for adding into the chaffles
- Shredded crab meat, 50 grams
- Garlic powder, 17 grams
- Bay seasoning, 17 grams
- For garnish:
- Chopped fresh cilantro, 20 grams
- Keto garlic mayonnaise, 34 grams
- Olive oil, 17 grams

Directions:

1. Heat your Chaffle maker.
2. Always remember you heat your Chaffle maker till the point that it starts producing steam.
3. Remove the egg whites in a bowl and beat them to the point that they become fluffy.
4. Beat the egg yolks in a separate bowl.
5. Add in the egg yolks in the egg whites and delicately mix them with a spatula.
6. Combine the eggs and cheese for the chaffle.

7. When your Chaffle maker is heated adequately, pour in the mixture.
8. Close your Chaffle maker.
9. Let your chaffle Cooking for five to six minutes approximately.
10. When your chaffles are done, dish them out.
11. Fry the shredded crab in olive oil until they are done.
12. Add the garlic powder and bay seasoning in the shredded crab.
13. Mix the garlic mayo and shredded crab together in a bowl.
14. Lay the crab mixture on the chaffle.
15. Roll your chaffle in the form of a taco.
16. Garnish the crab roll with the chopped cilantro.
17. Your dish is ready to be served.

Nutrition:

Protein: 48

Fat: 48

Carbohydrates: 4

Green Cayenne Chaffle

Preparation time: 10 minutes

Cooking Time: 14 Minutes

Servings: 2

Ingredients:

- 1 cup coconut flour
- 1/2 cup cream cheese, soft
- 1/2 cup coconut milk
- 1 tablespoon chives, chopped
- 1 tablespoon parsley, chopped
- 1 green chili pepper, minced
- 1/2 teaspoon cayenne pepper
- 1 teaspoon baking soda

Directions:

1. In a bowl, mi the eggs with the cream cheese, milk and the other ingredients and whisk well.
2. Preheat the Chaffle iron, pour 1/4 of the batter, close the Chaffle maker, Cooking for 10 minutes and transfer to a plate.
3. Repeat with the rest of the batter and serve.

Nutrition:

Calories 273

Fat 11.2

Fiber 3

Carbs 5.4

Protein 6

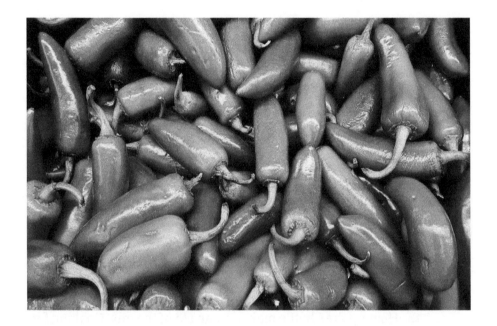

Hot Pesto Chaffles

Preparation time: 10 minutes

Cooking Time: 7 Minutes

Servings: 2

Ingredients:

- 1 cup almond milk
- 1 cup mozzarella, shredded
- 1 cup coconut flour
- 3 tablespoons basil pesto
- 1 teaspoon hot paprika
- 1 teaspoon chili powder
- 2 eggs, whisked
- 1 tablespoon ghee, melted
- 1 teaspoon baking soda

Directions:

1. In a bowl, mix the milk with the cheese, pesto and the other ingredients and whisk.
2. Heat up the Chaffle maker, pour 1/4 of the mix, Cooking for 7 minutes and transfer to a plate.
3. Repeat with the rest of the mix and serve.

Nutrition:

Calories 250

Fat 13 g

Fiber 4 g

Carbs 7.2 g

Protein 15 g

Tofu and Espresso Chaffles

Preparation time: 10 minutes

Cooking Time: 20 Minutes

Servings: 6

Ingredients:

- 2 cups almond flour
- 2 teaspoons cinnamon powder
- 1 tablespoon baking soda
- 1/2 teaspoon vanilla extract
- 11 ounces soft tofu, non GMO, crumbled
- 1/2 cup butter, melted
- 4 tablespoons stevia
- 1 tablespoon espresso

Directions:

1. In a bowl, mix the flour with baking soda and cinnamon and stir.
2. In your blender, mix tofu with espresso and the other ingredients, pulse well, add to the flour mix and stir until you obtain a batter.
3. Heat up the Chaffle iron; pour 1/6 of the batter and Cooking for 6 minutes.
4. Repeat with the rest of the batter and serve the chaffles cold.

Nutrition:

Calories 220

Fat 27 g

Fiber 2 g

Carbs 11 g

Protein 16 g

Cranberry Chaffles

Preparation time: 10 minutes

Cooking Time: 14 Minutes

Servings: 8

Ingredients:

- 1 and 3/4 cup almond flour
- 2 teaspoons baking powder
- 1/4 cup swerve
- 1/4 cup fat free Greek yogurt
- 1/4 cup coconut butter
- 2 eggs, whisked
- 2 tablespoons cream cheese, soft
- 1/2 cup cranberries
- 1 teaspoon vanilla extract

Directions:

1. In a bowl, combine the flour with the baking powder and the other ingredients and whisk.
2. Heat up the Chaffle iron; pour 1/8 of the batter, and Cooking for 5 minutes.
3. Repeat with the rest of the batter and serve the chaffles cold.

Nutrition:

Calories 200

Fat 20 g

Fiber 0 g

Carbs 8 g

Protein 17 g

Almond Butter Chaffles

Preparation time: 10 minutes

Cooking Time: 10 Minutes

Servings: 6

Ingredients:

- 2 eggs, whisked
- 2 tablespoons cream cheese, soft
- 1 cup almond butter
- 1 teaspoon almond extract
- 1/4 cup almond flour
- 2 tablespoons stevia
- 1/2 teaspoon baking soda

Directions:

1. In a bowl, combine the cream cheese with the almond butter and the other ingredients and whisk.
2. Heat up the Chaffle iron; pour 1/6 of the batter and Cooking for 7 minutes.
3. Repeat with the rest of the batter, divide the chaffles between plates and serve.

Nutrition:

Calories 140

Fat 12 g

Fiber 3 g,

Carbs 2 g

Protein 8 g

Avocado and Yogurt Chaffles

Preparation time: 10 minutes

Cooking Time: 5 Minutes

Servings: 4

Ingredients:

- 2 cups coconut flour
- 1/2 cup cream cheese, soft
- 1/2 cup yogurt
- 1/2 teaspoon baking soda
- 1 teaspoon baking powder
- 2 tablespoons stevia
- 2 eggs, whisked
- 3 tablespoons coconut oil, melted

Directions:

1. In a bowl, mix the flour with the yogurt and the other ingredients and whisk well.
2. Pour 1/4 of the batter in your Chaffle iron, close and Cooking for 5 minutes.
3. Repeat this with the rest of the batter and serve your chaffles right away.

Nutrition:

Calories 200

Fat 18 g

Fiber 2 g

Carbs 3 g

Protein 8 g

Chaffles and Raspberry Syrup

Preparation time: 10 minutes

Cooking Time: 20 Minutes

Servings: 4

Ingredients:

For Chaffles:

- 2 tablespoons stevia
- 1 and 1/4 cup coconut milk
- 1/4 cup coconut oil, melted
- 1/2 teaspoon almond extract
- 1 cup almond flour
- 1/2 cup coconut flour
- 1 and 1/2 teaspoons baking powder
- 1/4 teaspoon cinnamon powder

For the syrup:

- 1 and 1/3 cup raspberries
- 4 tablespoons lemon juice
- 1/2 cup water

Directions:

1. In a bowl, mix the stevia with the coconut oil, milk and the other ingredients except the ones for the syrup and whisk.
2. Pour 1/4 of the batter in your Chaffle iron, cover and Cooking for about 5 minutes.
3. Transfer to a plate and repeat with the rest of the batter.

4. Meanwhile, combine the raspberries with the lemon juice and the water, whisk heat up over medium heat for 10 minutes.

5. Drizzle the raspberry mix over your chaffles and serve.

Nutrition:

Calories 23

Fat 16 g

Fiber 5 g

Carbs 3 g

Protein 10 g

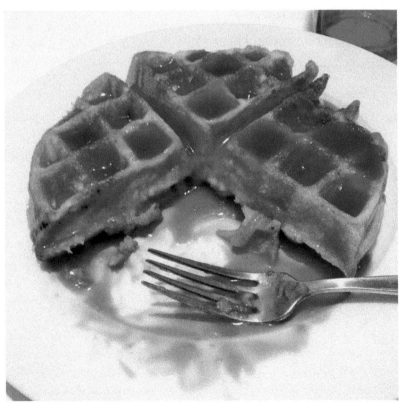

Pumpkin Seeds Chaffles

Preparation time: 6 minutes

Cooking Time: 5 Minutes

Servings: 4

Ingredients:

- 1 tablespoon coconut oil, melted
- 1 cup almond flour
- 1 egg, whisked
- 3 tablespoons cream cheese, soft
- 1 1/2cups almond milk
- 3 tablespoons stevia
- 2 tablespoons pumpkin seeds
- 1 teaspoon vanilla extract
- 1 teaspoon baking soda

Directions:

1. In a bowl, mix the melted coconut oil with the flour and the other ingredients and whisk well.
2. Heat up the Chaffle iron; pour 1/4 of the batter and Cooking for 5 minutes.
3. Repeat with the rest of the batter and serve the chaffles cold.

Nutrition:

Calories 220

Fat 14 g

Fiber 3 g

Carbs 3 g

Protein 9 g

Almond and Nutmeg Chaffles

Preparation time: 10 minutes

Cooking Time: 10 Minutes

Servings: 6

Ingredients:

- 1 cup coconut flour
- 1/2 cup cream cheese, soft
- 1/2 teaspoon nutmeg, ground
- 1 cup almond flour
- 3 eggs, whisked
- 1/4 cup almond butter, melted

Directions:

1. In a bowl, combine the flour with the cream cheese and the other ingredients and whisk.
2. Heat up the Chaffle iron; pour 1/6 of the batter and Cooking for 7 minutes.
3. Repeat with the rest of the batter and serve.

Nutrition:

Calories 200

Fat 18 g

Fiber 3 g

Carbs 4 g

Protein 8 g

Lemon Chaffle

Preparation time: 10 minutes

Cooking Time: 12 Minutes

Servings: 6

Ingredients:

- 1 cup almond flour
- 1 teaspoon baking powder
- 1/2 cup heavy cream
- 3 tablespoons cream cheese, soft
- 1 teaspoon baking soda
- 3 tablespoons coconut oil, melted
- 1 cup almond milk
- 3 tablespoons stevia
- 1/4 cup lemon juice

Directions:

1. In a bowl, combine the flour with the cream and the other ingredients and whisk well.
2. Heat up the Chaffle iron; pour 1/6 of the batter and Cooking for 7 minutes.
3. Repeat with the rest of the batter and serve cold.

Nutrition:

Calories 346

Fat 20 g

Fiber 1 g,

Carbs 6 g

Protein 9

Hot Pork Chaffles

Preparation time: 10 minutes

Cooking Time: 10 minutes

Serving: 4

Ingredients:

- 1 cup pulled pork, cooked
- 2 tablespoons parmesan, grated
- 2 eggs, whisked
- 2 red chilies, minced
- 1 cup almond milk
- 1 cup almond flour
- 2 tablespoons coconut oil, melted
- 1 teaspoon baking powder

Directions:

1. In a bowl, mix the pulled pork with the eggs, parmesan and the other ingredients and whisk well.
2. Heat up the Chaffle maker, pour 1/4 of the chaffle mix, cook for 8 minutes and transfer to a plate.
3. Repeat with the rest of the merge and serve.

Nutrition:

Calories 300

Fat 13 g

Fiber 4 g,

Carbs 7.2 g

Protein 15 g

Rhubarb Chaffles

Preparation time: 5 minutes

Cooking Time: 6 minutes

Serving: 3

Ingredients:

- 1/2 cup rhubarb, chopped
- 1/4 cup heavy cream
- 3 tablespoons cream cheese, soft
- 2 tablespoons almond flour
- 2 eggs, whisked
- 2 tablespoons swerve
- 1/2 teaspoon vanilla extract
- 1/2 teaspoon nutmeg, ground

Directions:

1. In a bowl, merge the rhubarb with the cream, cream cheese and the other ingredients and whisk well.
2. Heat up the Chaffle iron over high heat, pour 1/3 of the batter, close the Chaffle maker, cook for 5 minutes and transfer to a plate.
3. Repeat with the rest of the chaffle batter and serve.

Nutrition:

Calories 180,

Fat 4 g,

Fiber 1.2 g,

Carbs 2 g,

Protein 2.4 g

French Dip Keto Chaffle Sandwich

Preparation time: 5 minutes

Cooking Time: 12 minutes

Serving: 2

Ingredients:

- 1 egg white
- 1/4 cup mozzarella cheese
- 1/4 cup sharp cheddar cheese
- 3/4 tsp. water
- 1 tsp. coconut flour
- 1/4 tsp. baking powder
- Pinch of salt

Directions:

1. Set oven to 425 degrees.
2. Merge all of the ingredients in a bowl and stir to combine.
3. Set out 1/2 of the batter on the Chaffle maker and close lid. Set a timer for 4 minutes and do not lift the lid until the cooking time is complete. Lifting beforehand can cause the Chaffle keto sandwich recipe to separate and stick to the Chaffle iron. You have to let it cook the entire 4 minutes before lifting the lid.
4. Detach the chaffle from the Chaffle iron and set aside. Repeat the same steps above with the rest of the chaffle batter.

5. Seal a cookie sheet with parchment paper and place chaffles a few inches apart.
6. Attach 1/4 to 1/3 cup of the slow cooker keto roast beef from the following recipe. Make sure to drain the excess broth/gravy before adding to the top of the chaffle.
7. Attach a slice of deli cheese or shredded cheese on top. Swiss and provolone are both great options.
8. Set on the top rack of the oven for 5 minutes so that the cheese can melt. If you'd like the cheese to bubble and begin to brown, turn oven to broil for 1 min.
9. Enjoy open-faced with a small bowl of beef broth for dipping.

Nutrition:

Calories 118 kcal,

Carbohydrates 2 g,

Protein 9 g,

Fat 8 g,

Fiber 1 g

Double Choco Chaffle

Preparation time: 5 minutes

Cooking Time: 10 minutes

Serving: 2

Ingredients:

- 1 egg
- 2 teaspoons coconut flour
- 2 tablespoons sweetener
- 1 tablespoon cocoa powder
- 1/4 teaspoon baking powder
- 1 oz. cream cheese
- 1/2 teaspoon vanilla
- 1 tablespoon sugar-free chocolate chips

Directions:

1. Merge all the ingredients in a large bowl.
2. Mix well.
3. Pour half of the mixture into the Chaffle maker.
4. Seal the device.
5. Cook for 4 minutes.
6. Uncover and transfer to a plate to cool.
7. Repeat the procedure to make the second chaffle.

Nutrition:

Calories 171,

Total Fat 10.7 g,

Saturated Fat 5.3 g,

Cholesterol 97 mg,

Basil Cherry Tomato Chaffle

Preparation time: 5 minutes

Cooking Time: 12 minutes

Serving: 2

Ingredients:

- 1 egg, whisked
- 1/2 cup mozzarella, shredded
- 1 cup cherry tomatoes, cubed
- 2 tablespoons basil, chopped
- 2 tablespoons cream cheese, soft
- 1 teaspoon coriander, ground
- 1/2 teaspoon rosemary, dried
- 3 tablespoons tomato passata

Directions:

1. In a bowl, mix the egg with the cheese, cream cheese, coriander and rosemary and stir well. Preheat the Chaffle iron over high heat, pour half of the chaffle mix, cook for 6 minutes and transfer to a plate.
2. Redo with the rest of the batter, divide the tomatoes, tomato passata and rosemary over the chaffles and serve.

Nutrition:

Calories 252,

Fat 4.3 g,

Fiber 2.2 g,

Carbs 5 g,

Protein 11.2 g

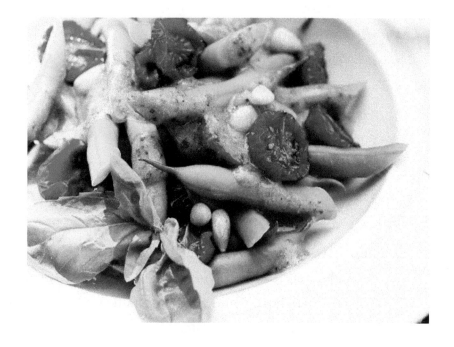

Green Chili Chaffle

Preparation time: 10 minutes

Cooking Time: 12 minutes

Serving: 6

Ingredients:

- 2 eggs, whisked
- 1 and 1/2 cup almond flour
- 1/2 cup cream cheese, soft
- 1/2 cup almond milk
- 1 teaspoon baking soda
- A pinch of salt and black k pepper
- 1/2 cup green chilies, minced
- 1 tablespoon chives, chopped

Directions:

1. In a bowl, mi the eggs with the flour, cream cheese and the other ingredients and whisk.
2. Preheat the Chaffle iron, pour 1/6 of the batter, close the Chaffle maker, cook for 8 minutes and transfer to a plate.
3. Redo with the rest of the batter and serve.

Nutrition:

Calories 265,

Fat 7 g,

Fiber 3 g,

Carbs 5.4 g,

Protein 6 g

Keto Fried Fish Chaffle Recipe

Preparation time: 25 minutes

Cooking Time: 20 minutes

Serving: 2

Ingredients:

- Mozzarella cheese, one cup
- Eggs, two for adding into the chaffles

For patties:

- Chopped fresh cilantro, 20 grams
- Egg, one
- Salt to taste
- Black pepper to taste
- Fish filet, 50 grams
- All-purpose flour, 17 grams
- Bread crumbs, 17 grams

For garnish:

- Avocado slices, half cup
- Lettuce leaf, two

For mayo sauce:

- Soy sauce, 17 grams
- Cilantro, 34 grams
- Swerve, 17 grams
- Mayonnaise, 5 grams

Directions:

1. Heat your Chaffle maker.
2. Always remember you heat your Chaffle maker till the point that it starts producing steam.
3. Remove the egg whites in a bowl and beat them to the point that they become fluffy.
4. Beat the egg yolks in a separate bowl.
5. Add in the egg yolks in the egg whites and delicately mix them with a spatula.
6. Combine the eggs and cheese for the chaffle.
7. When your Chaffle maker is heated adequately, pour in the mixture.
8. Close your Chaffle maker.
9. Let your chaffle Cooking for five to six minutes approximately.
10. When your chaffles are done, dish them out.
11. In the meanwhile, mix all the ingredients for the mayo sauce in a bowl.
12. Mix the ingredients for the fried fish.
13. Fry the fish in olive oil until they are done.
14. Lay a lettuce leaf on the chaffle, add the fried fish and place the avocado slices on top.
15. Pour the mayo sauce on top and close your sandwich.
16. Your dish is ready to be served.

Nutrition:

Calories 247

Fat 14g

Protein 9g

Carbs: 0.1

Italian Chicken and Basil Chaffles

Preparation time: 10 minutes

Cooking Time: 7-9 Minutes

Servings: 2

Ingredients:

Batter

- 1/2 pound ground chicken
- 4 eggs
- 3 tablespoons tomato sauce
- Salt and pepper to taste
- 1 cup grated mozzarella cheese
- 1 teaspoon dried oregano
- 3 tablespoons freshly chopped basil leaves
- 1/2 teaspoon dried garlic

Other

- 2 tablespoons butter to brush the Chaffle maker
- 1/4 cup tomato sauce for serving
- 1 tablespoon freshly chopped basil for serving

Directions:

1. Preheat the Chaffle maker.
2. Add the ground chicken, eggs and tomato sauce to a bowl and season with salt and pepper.
3. Add the mozzarella cheese and season with dried oregano, freshly chopped basil and dried garlic.

4. Mix until fully combined and batter forms.
5. Brush the heated Chaffle maker with butter and add a few tablespoons of the chaffle batter.
6. Close the lid and Cooking for about 7–9 minutes depending on your Chaffle maker.
7. Repeat with the rest of the batter.
8. Serve with tomato sauce and freshly chopped basil on top.

Nutrition:

Calories: 253

Fat: 17 g,

Protein: 11 g

Carbohydrates: 21 g

Fiber 2 g

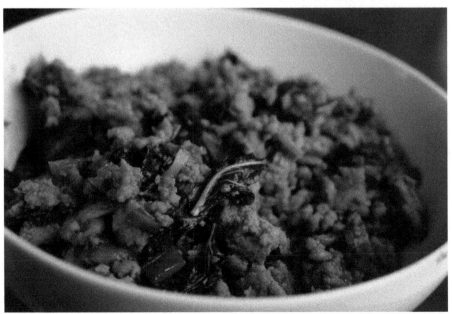

Beef Meatballs on Chaffle

Preparation time: 10 minutes

Cooking Time: 20 Minutes

Servings: 2

Ingredients:

Batter

- 4 eggs
- 21/2 cups grated gouda cheese
- 1/4 cup heavy cream
- Salt and pepper to taste
- 1 spring onion, finely chopped

Beef meatballs

- 1 pound ground beef
- Salt and pepper to taste
- 2 teaspoons Dijon mustard
- 1 spring onion, finely chopped
- 5 tablespoons almond flour
- 2 tablespoons butter

Other

- 2 tablespoons Cooking spray to brush the Chaffle maker
- 2 tablespoons freshly chopped parsley

Directions:

1. Preheat the Chaffle maker.

2. Add the eggs, grated gouda cheese, heavy cream, salt and pepper and finely chopped spring onion to a bowl.

3. Mix until combined and batter forms.

4. Brush the heated Chaffle maker with Cooking spray and add a few tablespoons of the batter.

5. Close the lid and Cooking for about 7 minutes depending on your Chaffle maker.

6. Meanwhile, mix the ground beef meat, salt and pepper, Dijon mustard, chopped spring onion and almond flour in a large bowl.

7. Form small meatballs with your hands.

8. Warmth the butter in a nonstick frying pan and Cooking the beef meatballs for about 3–4 minutes on each side.

9. Serve each chaffle with a couple of meatballs and some freshly chopped parsley on top.

Nutrition:

Calories: 159

Fat: 7 g

Protein: 9 g

Carbohydrates: 15 g

Fiber: 0.8 g

Leftover Turkey Chaffle

Preparation time: 10 minutes

Cooking Time: 7-9 Minutes

Servings: 2

Ingredients:

Batter

- 1/2 pound shredded leftover turkey meat
- 4 eggs
- 1 cup grated provolone cheese
- Salt and pepper to taste
- 1 teaspoon dried basil
- 1/2 teaspoon dried garlic
- 3 tablespoons sour cream
- 2 tablespoons coconut flour

Other

- 2 tablespoons Cooking spray for greasing the chaffle maker
- 1/4 cup cream cheese for serving the chaffles

Directions:

1. Preheat the Chaffle maker.
2. Add the leftover turkey, eggs and provolone cheese to a bowl and season with salt and pepper, dried basil and dried garlic.
3. Add the sour cream and coconut flour and mix until batter forms.

4. Brush the heated Chaffle maker with Cooking spray and add a few tablespoons of the chaffle batter.

5. Close the lid and Cooking for about 7–9 minutes depending on your Chaffle maker.

6. Repeat with the rest of the batter.

7. Serve with cream cheese on top of each chaffle.

Nutrition:

Calories: 74

Fat: 2 g

Protein: 4 g,

Carbohydrates: 10 g

Fiber: 0.2 g

Keto Lobster Roll Chaffle Recipe

Preparation time: 25 minutes

Cooking Time: 15 minutes

Serving: 2

Ingredients:

- Mozzarella cheese, one cup
- Eggs, two for adding into the chaffles
- Shredded lobster meat, 50 grams
- Garlic powder, 17 grams
- Bay seasoning, 17 grams
- For garnish:
- Chopped fresh cilantro, 20 grams
- Keto garlic mayonnaise, 34 grams
- Olive oil, 17 grams

Directions:

1. Heat your Chaffle maker.
2. Remove the egg whites in a bowl and beat them to the point that they become fluffy.
3. Beat the egg yolks in a separate bowl.
4. Add in the egg yolks in the egg whites and delicately mix them with a spatula.
5. Combine the eggs and cheese for the chaffle.
6. When your Chaffle maker is heated adequately, pour in the mixture.
7. Close your Chaffle maker.

8. Let your chaffle Cooking for five to six minutes approximately.

9. When your chaffles are done, dish them out.

10. Fry the shredded lobster in olive oil until they are done.

11. Add the garlic powder and bay seasoning in the shredded salmon.

12. Mix the garlic mayo and shredded lobster together in a bowl.

13. Lay the lobster mixture on the chaffle.

14. Roll your chaffle in the form of a taco.

15. Garnish the lobster roll with the chopped cilantro.

16. Your dish is ready to be served.

Nutrition:

Cal: 158

Total Fat: 15.2 g

Saturated Fat: 5.2 g

Cholesterol 269 mg

Sodium 178 mg

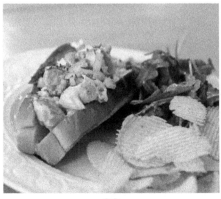

Keto Salmon Chaffle Tacos Recipe

Preparation time: 25 minutes

Cooking Time: 15 minutes

Serving: 2

Ingredients:

- Mozzarella cheese, one cup
- Eggs, two for adding into the chaffles
- Shredded salmon meat, 50 grams
- Garlic powder, 17 grams
- Bay seasoning, 17 grams
- For garnish:
- Chopped fresh cilantro, 20 grams
- Keto garlic mayonnaise, 34 grams
- Olive oil, 17 grams

Directions:

1. Heat your Chaffle maker.
2. Always remember you heat your Chaffle maker till the point that it starts producing steam.
3. Remove the egg whites in a bowl and beat them to the point that they become fluffy.
4. Beat the egg yolks in a separate bowl.
5. Add in the egg yolks in the egg whites and delicately mix them with a spatula.
6. Combine the eggs and cheese for the chaffle.

7. When your Chaffle maker is heated adequately, pour in the mixture.
8. Close your Chaffle maker.
9. Let your chaffle Cooking for five to six minutes approximately.
10. When your chaffles are done, dish them out.
11. Fry the shredded salmon in olive oil until they are done.
12. Add the garlic powder and bay seasoning in the shredded salmon.
13. Mix the garlic mayo and shredded lobster together in a bowl.
14. Lay the salmon mixture on the chaffle.
15. Roll your chaffle in the form of a taco.
16. Garnish the salmon taco with the chopped cilantro.
17. Your dish is ready to be served.

Nutrition:

Calories: 666

Fat: 55.2 g

Carbs: 4.8 g

Lettuce Chaffle Sandwich

Preparation Time: 9 minutes

Cooking Time: 5 minutes

Servings: 2

Ingredients:

- 1 large egg
- 1 tbsp. almond flour
- 1 tbsp. full-fat Greek yogurt
- 1/8 tsp. baking powder
- 1/4 cup shredded Swiss cheese
- 4 lettuce leaves

Directions:

1. Switch on your Mini Chaffle Maker.
2. Grease it with cooking spray.
3. Mix together egg, almond flour, yogurts, baking powder and cheese in mixing bowl.
4. Set 1/2 cup of the batter into the center of your Chaffle iron and close the lid.
5. Cook Chaffles for about 2-3 minutes until cooked through.
6. Repeat with remaining batter
7. Once cooked, carefully transfer to plate. Serve lettuce leaves between 2 chaffles.
8. Enjoy!

Nutrition:

Protein: 22

Fat: 66

Carbohydrates: 12

Vegetarian Chaffle Sandwich

Preparation Time: 9 minutes

Cooking Time: 8 minutes

Servings: 2

Ingredients:

Chaffle:

- 1 large egg (beaten)
- 1/8 tsp. onion powder
- 1 tbsp. almond flour
- 1/2 cup shredded mozzarella cheese
- 1 tsp. nutmeg
- 1/4 tsp. baking powder

Sandwich Filling:

- 1/2 cup shredded carrot
- 1/2 cup sliced cucumber
- 1/2 medium bell pepper (sliced)
- 1 cup mixed salad greens
- 1/2 avocado (mashed and divided)
- 6 tbsp. keto friendly hummus

Directions:

For the chaffle:

1. Plug the Chaffle maker to preheat it. Spray it with non-stick cooking spray.

2. Combine the baking powder, nutmeg, flour and onion powder in a mixing bowl. Add the eggs and mix.
3. Add the cheese and mix until the ingredients are well combined and you have formed a smooth batter.
4. Pour the batter into the Chaffle maker and spread it out to the edges of the Chaffle maker to cover all the holes on it.
5. Close the Chaffle lid and cook for about 5 minutes or according to Chaffle maker's settings.
6. After the cooking cycle, remove the chaffle from the Chaffle maker with a plastic or silicone utensil.

For the sandwich:

1. Add 3 tablespoons of hummus to one chaffle and spread with a spoon.
2. Fill another chaffle with one half of the mashed avocado.
3. Fill the first chaffle slice with 1/4 cup sliced cucumber, 1/2 cup mixed salad greens, 1/4 cup shredded carrot and one half of the sliced bell pepper.
4. Place the chaffle on top and press lightly.
5. Serve and enjoy.

Nutrition:

Fat: 22 g

Carbohydrate: 17.8 g

Sugars: 4.6 g

Protein: 11.3 g

Chaffle Cuban sandwich

Preparation time: 10 minutes

Cooking Time: 10 Minutes

Servings: 1

Ingredients:

- 1 large egg
- 1 Tbsp. almond flour
- 1 Tbsp. full-fat Greek yogurt
- 1/8 tsp. baking powder
- 1/4 cup shredded Swiss cheese

For The Filling:

- 3 oz. roast pork
- 2 oz. deli ham
- 1 slice Swiss cheese
- 3-5 sliced pickle chips
- 1/2 Tbsp. Dijon mustard

Directions

1. Turn on Chaffle maker to heat and oil it with cooking spray.
2. Beat egg, yogurt, almond flour, and baking powder in a bowl.
3. Sprinkle 1/4 Swiss cheese on hot Chaffle maker. Top with half of the egg mixture, and then add 1/4 of the cheese on top. Close and cook for 3-5 minutes, until golden brown and crispy.
4. Repeat with remaining batter.

5. Layer pork, ham, and cheese slice in a small microwaveable bowl. Microwave for 50 seconds, until cheese melts.
6. Spread the inside of chaffle with mustard and top with pickles. Invert bowl onto chaffle top so that cheese is touching pickles. Place bottom chaffle onto pork and serve.

Nutrition:

Carbs: 2 g

Fat: 24 g

Protein: 34 g

Calories: 352

Chicken Quesadilla Chaffle

Preparation time: 10 minutes

Cooking time: 14 minutes

Servings: 2

Ingredients:

- 1 egg, beaten
- 1/4 tsp. taco seasoning
- 1/3 cup finely grated cheddar cheese
- 1/3 cup cooked chopped chicken

Directions:

1. Preheat the Chaffle iron.
2. In a medium bowl, mix the eggs, taco seasoning, and cheddar cheese. Add the chicken and combine well.
3. Open the iron, lightly grease with Cooking spray and pour in half of the mixture.
4. Close the iron and cook until brown and crispy, 7 minutes.
5. Remove the chaffle onto a plate and set aside.
6. Make another chaffle using the remaining mixture.
7. Servings afterward.

Nutrition:

Calories 314

Fats 20.64g

Protein 16.74g

Simple Savory Chaffles

Preparation time: 6 minutes

Cooking Time: 8 Minutes

Servings: 4

Ingredients:

- 1 large organic egg, beaten
- 1/2 cup Cheddar cheese, shredded
- Pinch of salt and pepper

Directions:

1. Preheat a mini Chaffle iron and then grease it.
2. In a container, add all the fixings and beat until well combined.
3. Add half of the mixture into preheated Chaffle iron and Cooking for about 4 minutes or until golden brown.
4. Repeat with the remaining mixture.
5. Serve warm.

Nutrition:

Calories: 150

Net Carb: 0.

Fat: 11.9g

Saturated Fat: 6.7g

Carbohydrates: 0.6g

Dietary Fiber: 0g

Sugar: 0.3g

Protein: 10.2g

Parmesan Garlic Chaffle

Preparation time: 6 minutes

Cooking Time: 5 Minutes

Servings: 2

Ingredients:

- 1 Tbsp. fresh garlic minced
- 2 Tbsp. butter
- 1-oz cream cheese, cubed
- 2 Tbsp. almond flour
- 1 tsp. baking soda
- 2 large eggs
- 1 tsp. dried chives
- 1/2 cup parmesan cheese, shredded
- 3/4 cup mozzarella cheese, shredded

Directions:

1. Heat cream cheese and butter in a saucepan over -low until melted.
2. Add garlic and Cooking, stirring, for minutes.
3. Turn on Chaffle maker to heat and oil it with Cooking spray.
4. In a mixing container, whisk together flour and baking soda, then set aside.
5. In a separate container, beat eggs for 1 minute 30 seconds on high, then add in cream cheese mixture and beat for 60 seconds more.

6. Add flour mixture, chives, and cheeses to the container and stir well.
7. Add 1/4 cup batter to Chaffle maker.
8. Close and Cooking for 4 minutes, until golden brown.
9. Repeat for remaining batter.
10. Add favorite toppings and serve.

Nutrition:

Carbs: 5 g

Fat: 33 g

Protein: 19 g

Calories: 385

Chicken and Veggies Chaffles

Preparation time: 10 minutes

Cooking Time: 15 Minutes

Servings: 2

Ingredients:

- 1/3 cup Cooked grass-fed chicken, chopped
- 1/3 cup Cooked spinach, chopped
- 1/3 cup marinated artichokes, chopped
- 1 organic egg, beaten
- 1/3 cup Mozzarella cheese, shredded
- 1-ounce cream cheese, softened
- 1/4 teaspoon garlic powder

Directions:

1. Preheat a mini Chaffle iron and then grease it.
2. In a container, add all ingredients and mix until well combined.
3. Add 1/of the mixture into preheated Chaffle iron and Cooking for about 4-5 minutes or until golden brown.
4. Repeat with the remaining mixture.
5. Serve warm.

Nutrition:

Carbs: 4 g

Fat: 26 g

Protein: 26 g

Calories: 365

Aromatic Chicken Chaffles

Preparation time: 10 minutes

Cooking Time: 40 Minutes

Servings: 4

Ingredients:

- Chicken: 2 leg pieces
- Dried bay leaves: 1
- Cardamom: 1
- Whole black pepper: 4
- Clove: 4
- Water: 2 cups
- Eggs: 2
- Salt: 1/4 tsp.
- Shredded mozzarella: 1 cup
- Baking powder: 3/4 tbsp.

Directions:

1. Set a large pan and boil water in it
2. Add in chicken, bay leaves, black pepper, cloves, and cardamom and cover and boil for 20 minutes at least
3. Remove the chicken and shred finely and discard the bones
4. Preheat your mini Chaffle iron if needed
5. Mix all the remaining above-mentioned ingredients in a bowl and add in chicken
6. Grease your Chaffle iron lightly

7. Cook your mixture in the mini Chaffle iron for at least 4 minutes or till the desired crisp is achieved and serve hot

8. Make as many chaffles as your mixture and Chaffle maker allow

Nutrition:

Calories: 170

Fats: 13 g

Carbs: 2 g

Protein: 11 g

Lightning Source UK Ltd.
Milton Keynes UK
UKHW020645100621
385263UK00001B/164